Extraordinary Butterflies

Stories of resilience and hope from the EB community

Compiled by Vie Portland
Illustrations by Naomi and Charlotte

This book is dedicated to all of the Butterflies
who continue to survive and thrive
despite being told we shouldn't.

Contents

Foreword	6
A sweaty, painful, fairy tale	10
Finding sanctuary in community	18
My little fish	23
I'm a sister	26
When 2020 took my heart	27
The sunny side of EB!	35
Forever love	38
Love & hope	39
Don't wrap us in cotton wool	42
EB builds empaths	46
Butterfly girl	48
Dear diary…	52
When to wheelchair	54
It's the little things!	57
Eye of the tiger	60

Endless battle	64
The miracle and complexity of an EB baby	66
The EB armour	76
Love	79
Sports day	82
Oscar	86
An EB angel	88
EB	90
We celebrate a bruise!	91
Between the blisters	91
Learning from a mutation	94
As fragile as a butterfly	96
Living with EB	100
It's not all bad	103
Acknowledgements	105

Foreword

By Vie Portland

Back in 2016, my friend, James Dunn, and I talked about setting up a support group for people who live with EB. We wanted it to be a group where people felt safe to ask anything and where people could share celebrations that might not seem so big to those outside of the EB community. We wanted it to be a place for people who live with EB all of the time, whether that is the person with EB, their partners, parents or families.

Over the years, we've shared medical issues, practical issues around those things that only come up for people living with disabilities - such as school care plans, adapted driving, support, clothing advice, sock and shoe recommendations, dressings suggestions - and we've shared joyous events, such as a first, or a 21st, dance recitals, learning to drive, new partners, and new babies.

The group is what James and I set it up for and more.

In April 2023, I had an idea; I thought it would be wonderful to have a collection of pieces written by the UK EB community; stories that share the realities of living with the condition, that can help others in the worldwide community know they are not alone; that can be read by people new to the community, whether that's parents, friends, teachers, nurses, GPs, or charity staff. These are the stories you won't see in medical books or websites. These are our stories.

As you read through, you'll see the courage and the tenacity that we in the community share. We're frequently told what we shouldn't do; we frequently respond with, "watch me!" We have chosen to live alongside this condition, to bring it along for the ride. It causes constant pain, it disrupts plans, and it brings heartbreak, but we continue to live the best lives we can because, to paraphrase Peter Pan, to live is an awfully big adventure.

Personally, with my involvement in the community, watching how others are brought up, cared for, I wonder how different my life would be had I been born into a family like the wonderful families in this book and beyond, that did what they could to care for me and my disability. I wonder how I would have grown if I had I been allowed to use a pushchair for longer, been allowed a wheelchair, and been bought shoes and clothes more suitable for someone with EB skin. Honestly, I sometimes feel momentarily sad, because, from decades of neglect, my wonky body now lives with so many other chronic pain conditions. But, perhaps, had I not been in the family I was, I wouldn't be me, and maybe that me wouldn't have been so interested in learning so much about my condition and the other people that live with it; and that could have meant I wouldn't have got to know all of the incredible people I know in this community. And I wouldn't swap my EB family for anything.

James broke many of our hearts when he passed in April 2018, as he was a much-loved member of our community, and he is very much missed, but our Facebook group continues to thrive and grow, now with the fabulous Amy Price with me.

We're a rare breed. There's approximately 500,000 people in the world that have EB. That sounds like a big number but, to put it in context, there are more people that live in the city of Leicester in the UK than there are people with EB in the world. All of us featured here, all of us that live with EB 24/7, are the experts in this incredibly rare condition, and we hope we can make others be more aware of it.

In this book, we share our stories, in our own voices, so we can help others feel less alone and to help others feel they belong. We've written the book we needed.

Thank you for joining us.

Love, Vie

#ExtraordinaryButterflies

> "FEET, WHAT DO I NEED YOU FOR WHEN I HAVE WINGS TO FLY?"
>
> — Frida Kahlo

A sweaty, painful, fairy tale
By Vie Portland

EB has lived with me every minute since I was born.

It has caused pain, infection, exhaustion, and further disabilities.
It has taken too many people I love.
It has brought sadness and pain. Internally, externally, physically, emotionally.
And it's brought love and belonging.

The beginning

Apparently, I was born without skin on my bottom. Nothing was done. There was no known history of any skin conditions in my family, so I guess it was just considered an oddity.

One of my earliest memories is when I was around three. I don't remember grabbing the freshly poured coffee off of a table and accidentally pouring it over my chest. I don't remember being taken to A&E, or being wrapped in bandages. I do remember being pinned to a hospital gurney as medical staff peeled the sticky bandages from my chest, my skin tearing as they came away, me screaming in distress. It was "just" a bad burn, apparently.

Through childhood, I would have normal childhood wounds, with inexplicable extras. Grazes from falling over would get bigger with blisters. The wounds frequently looked far bigger than the accident warranted. I was told I was just being difficult, that my body was wrong.

My Mum walked everywhere. I'm the eldest but my next sibling was only 14 months younger; I remember walks where my sibling would be in the pushchair and I would be walking alongside, my little toddler legs struggling to keep up, my feet being so very sore. I was told I was lazy because I struggled to keep up; I was told I was whiny because I talked about the pain. I learned not to complain.

Both my parents loved the sun. From the age of 11 we would drive to Southern Spain for holidays. My siblings would spread out on the back seat and I would sit on the hump that used to be in the middle of the floor in cars; I was told that I had to look after them, that they needed more space than me, that, to be nice, I shouldn't complain about not having a seat; I definitely wasn't allowed to complain about the heat squished into that space, with no open window near; or the pain, because that would just be me moaning.

I struggled to be in the sun; if I sat in the tent, I was told off for being antisocial; when I sat in the sun and my skin blistered, I was attention-seeking. When my blisters got so big that I couldn't wear my shoes, I was told I was greedy for wanting a new pair. I remember the pain of being cut out of jelly shoes because my blisters had grown through the gaps and over the plastic; well, that was just rude of me.

My blistering skin was an inconvenience, it was my fault, I was doing it on purpose.

The rare times I was taken to see a GP, they looked at me with a confused expression. I was told my skin was too hard. I was told my skin was too soft. I was told I had eczema. I was told I sweated too much. Everything was my fault. No-one ever referred me to a dermatologist.

At school, I was embarrassed by my skin. I was embarrassed about all of me. I was told I was fat, ugly and worthless at home, so I assumed everyone else thought the same. I struggled with P.E., especially in the warmer months; that reiterated that I was fat and lazy. I got ridiculed for the way I walked when my feet were blistered.

But, at home, on my own in my bedroom, I could dance. With the cold breeze from the open window, without the fear of being judged, I would dance and sing. That was my place of joy. It hurt but it made me happy.

Once I left home, the embarrassment continued. I would never tell the families I worked for about the pain my skin caused. I would always hide my feet from boyfriends. It was only the children I cared for that I felt safe to have my feet out in front of; children just had their natural curiosity, asking me questions then getting distracted by something far more interesting.

Almost ten years after I left home, I worked up the courage to talk to a GP about my skin; I had to prepare myself for being told that it was all my fault again. But the GP didn't tell me it was my fault; they referred me to a dermatologist. And that dermatologist, at a big hospital in London, looked at my feet and said: "That's a prime example of Epidermolysis Bullosa Simplex Weber-Cockayne, you have there!"

Huh?!!

Apparently, my feet were such a good example of those words I had never heard before that he sent me to the hospital's photography lab to have photos taken for a medical journal!

He told me about the charity Debra, who raised awareness of people with my skin condition.

My skin condition.

It wasn't my fault. I hadn't done anything wrong.

I had a condition.

It took me several years before I could confidently talk about me having the condition, though; the years of being told all the horrible things made me think that no-one would like me if there was something else really wrong with me.

I started researching the condition and the charity. There were other people like me! I wasn't the freak of nature I was told I was!

I began to meet people with EB. For the first time in my life, at almost 30 years old, I felt I belonged somewhere. Oh my goodness! I cannot express how important that was!

I learned more about my condition, and the different other types of EB. I got involved in fundraising for the charity; I even gave talks about the condition. I remember my first talk for Debra; I was asked to speak to 25 women at a fitness event; now, I couldn't cope with people singing me "Happy Birthday", because that meant they were looking at me, so, to give a talk, that was HUGE! But I wanted to help, so I agreed.

I got to the venue and realised a 0 had been left off; it was 250 people! I wanted to run and hide but I had made a promise and I would keep it; I kept telling myself that I would never see these people again so, when I made a fool of myself, I could disappear from their lives.

But speaking to those women was a really important lesson; I realised that I am the expert in my condition. I realised that EB is so incredibly rare that the vast majority of people have never heard of it, so, whatever I told them, even if I said that the only thing that helped was sitting in a bath full of crisps while being covered in tomato ketchup, they wouldn't know whether it was right or wrong, because they knew nothing about it.

That was a very small, but very important, step to me being more confident in accepting my condition, and in talking about it.

With the growth of social media, more people with EB came into my life, from all over the world, many of whom became friends, some, very good friends.

I've had some wonderful weekends away with people with EB, and it's helped me accept my condition more fully; it's also helped in my growth in confidence.

The middle

Having grown up being told horrible things about how I looked, how I behaved, then going into relationships that reiterated those "facts", and having a condition that so few knew about, that had caused further chronic conditions, my mental and physical health plummeted in my mid-30s. I had a few very difficult years, where I felt I was really proving the messages I had been told: fat, ugly, worthless. What was the point of me?

Thankfully, I eventually realised that I had a choice: stay the same, end things, change things. I chose to change. I chose to challenge myself to live a happy life.

Part of that change was to stop seeing my family. I realised I was never going to fit, and that my mental health would not survive, that I would not survive, with them in my life.

Then I started challenging myself to do things I believed "someone like me" couldn't do.

First was dance! I was told as a child that no-one would want to look at me dancing so I didn't start classes until I was 15, when I could pay for them with money earned at my Saturday job, but, as the oldest in the class, I taught more than danced. But, I had set myself a challenge, and dance was the first thing. Not just dance; burlesque! I was even persuaded to perform! Me! Who hated to be looked at! And, from what was meant to be a once only performance, I went on to become an international performer! Audiences loved me! It was a big step to accepting who I was.

And accepting who I was also included accepting I had a disability.

I had no problems saying my friends with EB had a disability but, me? No! My strain of EB was nowhere near as bad as theirs, so to say I had a disability felt fraudulent. But, as I grew more confident with other aspects of my life, I realised that my experience of the condition shouldn't be based on how it compares with other people with EB, but to those people who don't live with it at all. And living with EB, at every level, is hard.

The now

Growing more confident with how I looked, and who I am, meant I became more accepting of my body, and of everything that made me wonky. And, from accepting it, I became astounded by it, very grateful for it, and, now, very proud of it.

My wonky body has survived horrors that many don't. My wonky body does everything it can to keep me alive, to keep me moving, even if those movements can only be small some days. My wonky body allows me to live a life I am happy in now. And my wonky body brought me the EB community, and I love them.

I used to be so embarrassed by sweating so much but, now, I am grateful my body does! Heat and friction are my main triggers for external blistering, so, by sweating, my body is working really hard to cool me down to attempt to minimise blistering. That's amazing!

I used to be really embarrassed by doing my constipated chicken walk when my feet were blistered; now, I am in awe that, despite all the pain my body is in, it keeps me going.

My EB affects every aspect of my life, in one way or another. I have to be careful about which shoes I wear, as I can't wear anything that makes my feet hot, or has too many straps. I have to think about the ground I walk on, as uneven and bobbly ground really hurts my feet. I have to think about how far I need to walk, and if it is worth the additional pain it will cause.

My hands shear, so I have to think about the things I pick up, the things I hold. Anything with ridges in, pens, cutlery, bottle tops, can tear my skin.

I have to think about my clothes. Anything too tight will cause friction and my skin will tear. I have to wear a vest under my bra, as the skin under my breasts tears easily and is especially prone to infection. I have to wear pants that are on the bigger side so my knicker line doesn't tear. I always wear shorts under my dresses so my thighs don't blister. I have to be careful with fabrics and labels, as I itch all of the time (a side effect for many of us with EB) and some fabrics will exacerbate that, causing more of my skin to breakdown. The extra layers are great in the colder months but, in the warmer months when you're battling to keep cool to avoid more blistering, it's difficult.

I have to think carefully about everything I eat because so many foods cause my mouth and throat to tear and blister. I can't eat anything spicy, peppery, or acidic (spicy is obvious, but many salad leaves are too peppery to eat, and the majority of fruits are acidic), nor anything too hard, such as boiled sweets, or too sharp, like crisps. Thankfully, I have found that Montezuma's Giant Chocolate Buttons are just the right size and temperature to sit inside a blistered cheek, and that M&S marshmallows are great to pop a blister in my throat.

And there's so much more. More things to be aware of. More pain to live with.

But, for me, there is also joy.

The happily ever after

I now give talks in school assemblies and at events about living with hidden disabilities and being more inclusive. I love raising awareness of EB, and encouraging people to see beyond what is right in front of them. I know I have made people more aware, and I know I have made a difference to all of the people that hadn't felt brave enough to talk about their hidden disabilities before, but now know, because of hearing me speak, that their voice, their story, deserves to be heard.

I love how me being confident enough to talk about living with hidden disabilities has made so many aware that not all disabilities are the same.

And I love that I have the EB community in my life.

I have been asked over the years why I remain so involved in the community when I have lost so many people I love to it, when there are times that survivor's guilt adds to my tears, and I say to them that meeting people with EB was the first time I felt accepted; that loving people with EB, and by being loved by them, is the first time I felt loved; and I tell them that they are my home.

"*THE MEASURE OF A MAN, OR WOMAN, IS NOT SO MUCH WHAT THEY HAVE ACCOMPLISHED, THOUGH THAT HAS WEIGHT. IT OFTEN IS MUCH MORE THAN WHAT THAT MAN OR WOMAN HAS OVERCOME TO ACCOMPLISH WHAT THEY HAVE.*"

— Leif Gregersen

Finding sanctuary in community

By Anonymous

"I'm honestly so proud of him and the young man he has become. EB will always be a part of him, but he said, 'I won't let it beat me'.

I had my son at 17. Here, I share the perspective of being a young Mum to a child with EB Simplex.

When the midwife came to visit me after my son's birth I remember her commenting on his hands and feet and saying she thought he had hand, foot and mouth disease. Soon, every page in my baby's 'red book' mentioned blisters on his hands and feet.

Every doctor, health visitor or professional involved mentioned it or commented on it but no-one ever seemed to provide any answers. He was often misdiagnosed, only to be told later: "No, actually it's not that."

As a young Mum, I felt overwhelmed. I wondered what was wrong with my baby, and why couldn't I get answers? I felt judged by professionals because of my age, and always felt that I had done something wrong to cause this – but, I didn't know what. I don't have any family history of EB that I'm aware of, but I don't know all of my family history on my father's side.

To me, my baby was perfect; I couldn't understand why everyone was making a big deal out of his blistering.

When he started to crawl, however, his hands started to get sore and I could see he was in pain as his skin would come away from his hands. I broke down to the doctor and begged him to help us figure this out. He said to me: "I don't know what is wrong with your son, I have no idea." He was the first person that admitted he didn't have a clue. He told me that he had never seen this before and agreed to refer my son to the dermatologist at Birmingham Children's Hospital. At last, we were going to get some idea of what it could be.

I remember walking into the children's hospital in Birmingham and seeing the nurse. Answering her questions, I told her how he would get blisters and they would be so big, then they would burst and be really sore like open wounds. I told her everything, like how they would heal and then come back again.

It sounds silly, but for the first time I felt like I wasn't being judged and that she actually understood. I remember that she looked at the other nurse and said, "are you thinking what I'm thinking, that he has EB Simplex?" I had never heard of this before and asked questions which she answered. Then he was taken for a biopsy and blood test. I also had to have blood tests too. She wrote the name Epidermolysis Bullosa Simplex on a piece of paper and told me not to google it - which I did, of course, as soon as I left, and, yes, I panicked.

Part of me was relieved because for the first time someone seemed to understand what I was saying and what I was going through, but another part of me was also sad as I was expecting them to just give me a magic cream to make it go away. My son was given a clinical diagnosis which was later confirmed through genetic testing on my side.

I remember the day he was first diagnosed, leaving the hospital armed with leaflets, dressings, creams and needles. As a young Mum, I remember feeling so overwhelmed. I was sad because my boy couldn't play without his hands being sore and when he got older he couldn't wear normal shoes as his feet would blister.

I remember now all the times when he was at primary school that I had to carry him from the car to the classroom because his feet were so sore that he couldn't put shoes on. When he became too big to carry he would stay at home on days when he couldn't walk. Because he couldn't go to school, I would take the day off work and we would stay home together.

Every morning and night I would lance his blisters and apply the dressings, it became a part of our normal daily routine. I remember times when he cried in pain, and I wished more than anything I could take away his pain. Sometimes he would say to me, "why do I have to have this Mum", and it broke my heart that I couldn't fix it. My son wanted to climb and play like the other children his age.

Life was difficult because I was working full time, studying and I also had another child now who did not have EB. I was so overwhelmed at times but reminded myself that it was only EB Simplex and lots of EB children have it much worse. I don't know if it's because I was a young parent and wanted to prove myself, but I was often too proud to ask for help or admit I was struggling.

When my son was around 10 or 11, I went for his routine review meeting at the children's hospital and my sister came with me, she helped me tell the EB nurse everything. The fact that he couldn't wear shoes, the fact that he would stay home because he couldn't walk on his feet for long and so we would often cut days out short, how when it was hot the blisters became much worse, and how he struggled to write at school because the pen rubbed. The nurse was so lovely and she helped me so much. She was assertive with me in a kind and humorous way and told me off for not asking for help all this time. I remember I said something like, "but he only has the mild version and I feel bad for complaining when there are children so much worse off". She said that I shouldn't think like that and just because there are worse kinds it doesn't mean that we shouldn't ask for support too as it's important that all children are supported.

The nurse put me in touch with the patient support charity Debra. She also helped me to get a wheelchair. I was so against this at first because he can physically walk, but she told me that it was only for when we went on days out so he could rest his feet for a while and we wouldn't have to leave early. She gave me some cooling dressings that we can put in the fridge for hot days, and she spoke to his school so he didn't have to wear school shoes and they made him a medical pass so he could leave lessons if needed. We also had a disabled parking badge so that he didn't have to walk so far. It was this combination of lots of small things that made a big difference!

I was so glad that I swallowed my pride and asked for support. I also decided to join Vie's group on Facebook that Debra had told me about and I found a community of others that also understood what we were going through. They knew about Bullen healthcare, Mepilex and sharps' boxes – it was like hearing people speaking a language that only I had known for so long and I didn't feel alone anymore on this journey. I remember one time a stranger on the group posted us some dressings to try and it was the kindest thing ever and I will always remember that.

Over the years, my son's EB became easier to manage as he knew how to care for it and would learn what his limits were so as not to make it worse. I think he just accepted that he couldn't do these things and became okay with it. For example, when his younger brother went climbing and he couldn't join in this made me feel sad but my boy said, "it's okay Mum, it hurts my hands and will make my EB bad so I'll just watch".

My son is now 17. The same age I was when I had him. He is at college and has a volunteer job for a charity. He is into rock music and plays the guitar which is something I never ever thought he would ever be able to do with EB. It amazes me. He said because he uses a plectrum and because he's pressing with the tips of his fingers he can play in a way that prevents/minimises blisters as it doesn't cause much friction. Of course, blisters do come sometimes, but he knows to stop and take a break. He's really good at playing.

He still struggles with days when his feet are sore and the skin has come away and I know sometimes he is uncomfortable, but he doesn't let it get him down anymore. I'm honestly so proud of him and the young man he has become. EB will always be a part of him, but he said, "I won't let it beat me".

> "WOUNDS ARE OFTEN THE OPENINGS INTO THE *BEST* AND MOST *BEAUTIFUL* PARTS OF US"
>
> – David Richo

My little fish

By Star Keeble
(Age 14)

My little fish who has EB,
My little fish nicknamed by me,
My little fish who loves dogs,
My little fish also likes frogs.

My little fish you have your scar,
My little fish your big sisters Charlie and Star,
My little fish you shine so bright,
My little fish you have so much might.

My little fish sometimes you may be in pain,
My little fish you are the main,
My little fish you also have wounds,
My little fish you make the cutest little sounds.

My little fish loving and kind,
My little fish her heart not blind,
My little fish is a bit bombastic,
My little fish is extra fantastic.

My little fish likes to watch TV,
My little fish loves bowbow's tea,
My little fish makes people smile,
My little fish I ran 26 miles.

My little fish although EB has no cure,
My little fish your heart is so pure,
My little fish you are not feeble,
That is purely because you are a Keeble.

My little fish I love to bits,
My little fish likes to eat ritz,
My little fish loves to play,
If she could, she would play all day.

My little fish I would do anything for,
My little fish who I adore,
My little fish likes to doodle,
My little fish would love a poodle.

My little fish you are our ray of sunshine,
My little fish your smile is so divine,
How I'm so lucky to have you,
You are the real-life version of Boo.

My little fish very, very cute,
My little fish could play a flute,
My little fish I love you so much,
I love you that much that I would tell you in Dutch.

By your big sister, Star xxx

Inspired by Ray Keeble, my sister

I'm a sister

By Charlie Keeble
(Age 9)

I'm a sister of a butterfly baby, she flies to me with butterfly love.

I'm a sister to the unknown, where dark skies can be above, but bright skies peer through.

I'm a sister that lives a war. In the battlefields I see a sunflower; right there is my sunshine, my baby sister.

I'm a sister to a baby blister, her blisters are sore and she cries. Her sadness turn to laughter as I pull silly monkey faces.

I'm a sister to a EB baby, her love makes me happy. EB or not, I love her so much. She is my sunshine, my only sunshine.

Inspired by Ray Keeble, my sister

When 2020 took my heart

By Danielle Keeble

Being pregnant is a joyful time. Being pregnant is a seed growing into a flower.

Being pregnant and enduring a horrendous loss, which no words can describe, the pain rips through, like a thousand knives; my daddy had gone to the world unknown.

Being pregnant with a darkness so great the joy is slowly disappearing, hoping there will be some light somewhere, riddled with grief, a burden untold in a hidden corner so that the children don't see.

Being pregnant with uncertain times, a plague upon us, a storm spiralling out of control, lightning hit us once already, and the fear it was coming again, wind blowing in all directions - how do I hold on when so scared of what's to come.

Being in labour frozen solid, nowhere to turn, no comfort, no joy... being frightened, wearing a gas mask like I was in the war, being in the peak of the plague in a place that everyone wanted to avoid, the same place my daddy took his last breath two months prior, panic setting in, how do I do this alone?

Being in labour feeling very alone, no care, no compassion, because every patient is treated like they are contagious, a big red X, stay clear do not approach was how I felt I was looked upon, no midwife would come near, with their back towards me by the door watching my contractions on a screen.

Being in labour, 28hrs in and things are progressing, reading one barcode on the bed for hours and hours, the pain was too much, but I have to find the strength.

Being in labour and its time - 36hrs have gone by - to meet our third child, this baby who will soon rock my world, here comes the storm again, my heart was already broken into a thousand pieces, surely no more devastation.

Being a mummy to a newborn, my seed has flowered.

Being handed my bundle of joy, the baby who I had carried and walked with me throughout the darkest times, I hold her, looking at her I notice things no-one else did, a hole... how is there a hole in my baby's hand? I look to the side of her and there is the shock of my life. I see red, lots of red... where has her skin gone? I start to panic, looking at anyone who will make eye contact with me, no words coming from my mouth but I am screaming so loud inside. Why is no-one looking, I need help.

The time is ticking by, but time has stood still, loads of doctors and nurses coming and going so fast, but they're in slow motion.

No-one knew what was upon us, being asked if mummy and daddy were related, because they didn't understand our baby - words I'll never forget.

Different departments coming to see our baby, like she is a piece in a museum, nurses taking photos like she is famous, famous for being skinless, but not once knowing what effect this was having on mummy and daddy; no-one cared, no-one asked us, we just felt that we were a circus show, all the lights beaming at us... but they were burning through us, like we were above and the area was a mist, slow motion, yet high speed.

Being a mummy to a baby who couldn't be held and couldn't be dressed is not natural, thinking what were we going to do...

Not knowing what we were dealing with, and the professionals didn't know either, but we found power, strength and courage to protect this fragile being from a painful guessing game of being rubbed, poked and pricked.

The skin was coming away before our eyes, rubbing to find a vein... "Stop," I shouted, knowing this was not right, the pain ripping through my soul and I couldn't take the pain away from my baby, I couldn't help my baby.

Two days old and already been through so much pain, the real professionals are coming, nurses from Great Ormond Street Hospital... when you hear those words, the surreal world is becoming real. "Is this happening?". What are they going to tell us?

They're here... with a whole-hearted smile, care and compassion across their faces, you know this look isn't good as much as it is comforting. An overload of a world we had never heard of, not grasping any words coming out, hearing what they were saying, but rejecting every word... the room seemed to be getting smaller, and smaller.

Then the nurses took our baby and told us to stay there, but against their advice I went with her... a biopsy? What's a biopsy for, did she have cancer? My mind went into overdrive, thinking all things but coming to no conclusion.

Not knowing how a biopsy was done, I'd never had to think about it, all I could do was hum to her with tears rolling down my face as I cradled over the top of her, I was so broken and at that point I felt I couldn't take much more. But more was to come, like a tsunami, one after another.

Going into the mother's room after, screaming at my dad "how could you leave me, why would you leave me now at my absolute lowest, my darkest time when I need you most". Selfishly; it was no fault of his. Being so angry, scared, irritated, exhausted, lost and every emotion you could think of - they were all rumbling inside me. I went back into our room where my baby was calm, sleeping... how can you be sleeping after that, the biopsy? I am in such a state... this baby is already stronger than me, will we help each other through this? Is she already carrying me? Teaching me?

I went outside to call my mum, with such despair I sobbed down the phone to her, she couldn't come to me because of the pandemic, how cruel this all was, she is a mum and a nan and being so torn for a second time in the space of three months of disaster was her deepest darkness, but she had my other children to care for and keep safe. She told me "everything will be just fine, your daddy is beside you and will keep you safe, he will guide you and protect you". Even though I told her what was happening and how bad my baby was, she knew that my baby was wrapped in angel wings and healing would start soon. I knew this would also break her, but there was nothing either of us could do to comfort each over, we had to care for the children we had.

Being a mummy to a beautiful baby girl who had my heart gripped tight, for the eight days we were in hospital was the most horrendous... she wore no clothes, wrapped in bandages, hooked up to two drips, she had an infection, a serious infection to her skin, with blood in her stools for six weeks because she was on such strong antibiotics.

The hospital didn't know how to deal with EB, uneducated in it, which made our world very difficult; we had to learn very quickly what was best for our baby, we became the experts overnight.

Being in hospital in the heat of the pandemic, scared witless, a vulnerable baby, was the last thing needed at this time, baby being tested for covid, knowing the swabs would cause her damage but they still did it. Why would they test her, she had just been born, born with missing skin, they could see, but they still swabbed her creating more sores, her mouth was already in a bad way, blisters on her gums, white pressure areas of scarring in her mouth and they still swabbed her.

The Great Ormond Street nurses came back to the hospital to tell us it was EB, I had no idea what this is about, I was told not to Google it, so I was in the midst of a blur.

They couldn't work out the baby's type as she wasn't straight forward... 3 types they thought she had: junctional, simplex and kindler syndrome, they told us she could die before she was two years old if she had a certain type, and said they have to do more testing.

We were told we may have to wait for weeks, months, even years for the testing. Our hearts and souls were shattered. Looking at baby Ray thinking how can this little beautiful baby leave me, starting to doubt if God really existed because if that were the case, why did he take my dad, and let my baby be born this way; no baby deserves this.

Being a mummy and still in the hospital, the moment EB hit me... when a nurse couldn't get the sticker tape of the cannula off the baby's skin, she was using the adhesive remover wipes, and it was taking too long, maybe she thought they weren't working, but little by little the stick was coming away, the nurse must have lost patience and decided to pull the tape without the wipe, my eyes burned with anger, I felt I could have done some serious harm because my emotions were out of this world. She had just caused my baby severe pain, the tape pulled my baby's skin off to the flesh, two inches of it, and she screamed in pain. And the nurse had no remorse for what she had just done. This was the second time a nurse caused my baby unnecessary pain, knowing they were doing it, and it was the last time this was going to happen... I took control, we became the nurses in that room.

Baby became jaundiced and had to be under a lamp with eye patches on. I believe this dried out some of her wounds, as she laid there sometimes calm but mostly screaming because she didn't like it or was in pain, we kept getting told off for taking her out of the incubator, but she was in such distress.

My mind was a whirlwind, how could this be, I've never heard of this or even seen it... how does this condition exist? It's so, so cruel and horrific. Children suffering this way, what a crushing reality hit I had.

Being a mummy and finally being able to take my baby daughter home.... it's meant to be the most exciting feeling, but it was the scariest feeling I have ever had, even though we took over the baby's care during our stay in hospital, the feeling of no emergency services to hand was a horrendous thought. What happens if she gets another infection? What happens if she needs serious medical help? How will we cope? My baby had serious open wounds from her waist down, now I am going to be her mummy, her nurse, her doctor and her support line... I was scared.

How do we take her home? I can't strap her in a car seat, and I can't leave her naked..... looking back at it, it was like the film *Fast & Furious: Tokyo Drift*, where they are looking down from a building and life down below is moving so fast, cars and people rushing around, then fast forward again.

We packed up and got the baby ready for a massive step in her life, a transition I was uneasy about, her clothes. We put them on for the first time, nothing I chose for her before she was born, her welcome to the world stuff or her frilly outfit, it was a white baby grow turned inside out, and I wrapped her in my dad's towel to protect her, placed her in the car seat and strapped the straps loosely.

We were ready and discharged... as we got out of the lift of the hospital, one of the nurses who had been seeing to our baby told us the baby's clothes were inside out... Those words gave me the confidence to walk out of that hospital, they had no clue, even with some firsthand experience.

We are home, it feels strange, quiet but almost a sense of calm... we survived the time in the hospital.

Everything was clean and ready and that gave me the time to learn how to be a mum to a special baby girl. I felt like a new mum again, even with two older girls this was far different from what I knew. So many medical items, all of her new baby creams, powders, wipes, nappies got packed away, along with most of her new beautiful baby clothes because she couldn't use or wear them, replaced with medical creams, dressings and lots of baby grows. How strange it felt to remove all of those items I got excited buying, getting ready for when she was born.

Sleeping now, a sleep full of worry... I used to lay awake, checking she was breathing and if I couldn't see her chest moving, I would nudge her. Having a baby who may not make it, not understanding the condition well, you naturally think all sorts, the most extreme things, darkest things. I would physically shake my head at times to remove the thoughts that were passing through my mind, I couldn't stop thinking of the worse.

The Great Ormond Street Hospital EB nurses were coming to our home, two weeks after we got home with our baby, they were coming to tell us if our baby was going to live... this day was dark, emotions unexplainable, no words spoken beforehand, the house so quite you could hear yourself breathing... They are here, Janet and Katie, with their comforting smiles and care, they said "it's good news, she doesn't have the two types that are life limiting, but she does still show a multi type and we woud have to wait for the full tests to come back, which could take up to a year" they explained. Her life could be still limited due to certain things that come with EB: infections, long wound healing, cancer and in baby Ray's case muscular dystrophy because part of her EB came with a mutation from the plectin gene (PLEC) pyloric atresia. The GOSH nurses assured us they will be there for us all the way and got Debra involved, the charity that supports EB.

After the nurse went it was all a blur, still not fully understanding what EB really was.

But being introduced to Debra, and being given our own personal lifeline through a member of Debra's support team: Amelia, who was absolutely amazing. She guided us through thick and thin, put us in touch with other services that could help, her understanding and compassion on how we were feeling as a family was out of this world, we weren't alone.

Being a mummy to my other two girls, not being able to see them this whole time, 10 days away from them while we were in hospital and not even a cuddle from them. It was two more weeks after coming home from hospital as I had to isolate away from them due to Covid and being in hospital. God, I missed them both more than words could speak, how having a baby with additional needs can pull you away from your other children, being put in that situation where you have to make that choice.

The time has come, the girls and my mum can finally meet baby Ray. We are off to my mum's house, a feeling of relief, excitement, worry and joy. Their faces when they see her, they know she is poorly and can't hold her very much, but their understanding as children was out of this world, care, compassion and love already instilled.

Being a mummy after this journey, things are starting to fall into place, finding our feet in a changed life, because this is a new world, the life we once knew has gone, things are very different. Riddled with grief and having this butterfly baby was a lot to deal with and even though I was in a very dark place we had to make it right for the girls.

A year later we finally got baby Ray's full results back. She was diagnosed with ebs-pa, which is epidermolysis bullosa pyloric atresia, which was a blow. To understand what this was, it took a long time for me to figure out and understand this gene. She is also recessive so my partner and I should have both carried the gene, but I didn't; baby Ray mutated her own version - what are the odds of that? We had never heard of EB, even though my partner carries the gene, it has never come out in his family.

Days, weeks, months and years have gone by, the hurdles we as a family have had to overcome, every day is different, finding out how to dress difficult wounds, adapting to different clothes, nappy changes are different, so much to take on board.

Being a mummy and having to go back to work after all of this. I did not want to go, I didn't want to go into people's houses because I was petrified of the virus and bringing it home to my family and the vulnerabilities in the house. And leaving the baby was so hard but my mum took over her care in the day... we found a way of making this terrible situation work, both riddled with grief and having to still run day-to-day life, normality as much as possible for the children's sake.

Being a mummy and being told your baby might not make her first birthday, now she's having her third birthday, and such a beautiful Ray of sunshine she is, she took her boo pars (grandad) name, even though he just missed her birth he walks with her every second of the day, RayRay will be forever protected and shielded in his wings.

It was once said to me, "You know when you're still alive because of the pain you're feeling." Even though I felt motionless throughout this time, I knew I was still alive. There is only so much a person can cope with, and epidermolysis bullosa takes you far beyond those coping levels, because you cannot take your baby's pain away. Can you imagine watching your child being tortured daily... no parents or grandparents would ever like to see a baby or child in this much pain. Unfortunately this is what families with EB children see every single day.

It is a heartbreaking disease, it's so very cruel and most of all it's absolutely devastating for the children suffering with it.

Today RayRay is a beautiful bonny little girl, she has her sores and blisters and goes through stuff I wish she didn't have to, but she loves to play, swim, and go to the park. She has the biggest love for her family, and she is the weirdest, funniest human being ever, with her big beautiful blue eyes and her contagious smile.

We as a family are so blessed to have her with us today. 2020 brought catastrophic events to our door, like the grim reaper was hanging above, we couldn't stop what was unfolding.

One day RayRay will have her own story to tell, but for now I'm doing it for her.

The Sunny Side of EB!

By Krystal Prescod

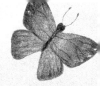

When we hear about EB, we most commonly hear about the medical side, the pain, the restrictions on life, so instead, I wanted to mention some of the Sunny Side of EB!

From my beginning into my early teens, I didn't even have a diagnosis! Which meant, I also did not have any treatment. As a result of this, I had great problem solving skills from my early years! It never occurred to my parents or me when I was old enough to even give me paracetamol for the pain. I found out that minty foot lotions would help ease the pain. So my Mum and Gran would always buy me nice minty foot lotions, and I would happily massage them into my feet, being careful to avoid any open wounds. I enjoyed putting those minty lotions on my feet, which also formed one of my first mindfulness experiences. I also expanded my problem solving skills as I was trying to find new ways to lance the blisters more effectively and without them refilling (I can dream can't I? lol).

During high school PE classes, when everyone griped about having to run for the first 20 minutes, I always got to sit out, unless I didn't like the main activity. The times were a little different in the early 2000's, so I was made to either do the activity or run, even on the days that I should have been exempt from both. I focused on being happy to skip the run, or activity that I didn't like.

When I did my Applied Business Technology and Legal Administrative courses in Canada, I received a $2,000 grant from the government, solely because of my EB, which was definitely a great blessing!

Due to the EB, I don't have to stand in the long queues!! I was very grateful for this at Disneyland California, and Paris! I have also been given free and heavily discounted entry into many tourist attractions in Europe along with priority entry.

As I grew up more, and started meeting other people out in the real world with their various disabilities, I had a greater understanding and empathy for what they may be battling.

I found that I have a particularly high empathy for those with foot pain, such as my dear husband. He has flat feet, and some other skin issues on his feet, which he has been neglectful until it causes him pain. Since I am always having to take care of my "little feeties" I have also been encouraging him to take care of his better, which has greatly improved his feet over all.

One of the greatest parts of having EB has come to me since moving her to the UK, is meeting and forming my own little EB family! I have absolutely loved meeting more of the community at the Member's Weekend and the Parliament Reception. I have loved getting to be a part of DebRA and interacting with them. These people, they know who they are, have brightened up my life!!

In the end, it comes down to this: EB is all I know. I have an amazing life that I am thankful for and EB has not stopped me from anything that I truly wanted or was meant for me, and there are some wonderful things that I may not have had without EB.

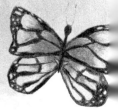

> "IT'S **WHO WE ARE** AND **WHAT WE DO** THAT MATTERS; THE REST IS JUST FANCY PACKAGING"
>
> – Vie Portland

Forever love

By Hon Lee-Davis, for Rachel

It's amazing how life turns out
Without a doubt
Someone above is watching over us
With all the signs that fate sowed
And the arrow from Cupid's bow
You opened up and let your love show

Straight to my heart from yours
The first time I embraced you
I felt like coming home
Don't you know how complete that makes me feel?
When I know you're the one

When I look into your eyes
I see forever love
You are like an angel sent from up above
For a future of ever-lasting love

Every time you hold me close I feel
So warm and so at peace
Even the touch from your lips
Makes my heart skip a beat

Without pain and without worries
That's how your love distracts me
As my soul travels with yours to infinity
My love for you goes beyond eternity

The things that love do
Makes me write love poems just for you
With all my heart I give to you
This is how much I love you

Love & hope

By Rachel Lee-Davis

I met Hon back in 2009. He had such a zest for life, he was truly inspiring to meet and didn't let anything hold him back, especially his EB. We immediately hit it off, became very good friends and would talk for hours on end. I had never met anyone like Hon. We just clicked. He was my missing piece of jigsaw. Those deep brown eyes; I could see into his soul, he just shines. We fell in love. We got married a year later and the rest is history!

Hon is highly intelligent and went to university to achieve his degree. He also did a Skydive in 2005 and is absolutely fearless. He really is the bravest person I know.

Hon has Junctional Non-Herlitz/Intermediate form of EB. He is 44 years young. There is no cure. Life is never boring, that's for sure; EB certainly makes life unpredictable. We spend hours and hours doing baths/dressings/creams/popping blisters daily. EB is 24/7, 365 days of the year - it is relentless. We call it the beast of EB.

Hon's attitude is you always have to control EB, otherwise it will control you.

Hon had the world's first kidney transplant with EB in 2012. Eleven years on, thankfully he is still going strong. It gave us our freedom back having spent over two years on home haemodialysis. We started to travel again and we make sure we enjoy every moment we have together.

Due to the kidney transplant, Hon has to take several immunosuppressants. These have caused three episodes of squamous cell carcinoma which we are still battling together to this day. He is also at very high risk of sepsis due to the extent of his wounds head to toe. We stay as positive as we can and we face every challenge head on together.

The corneal abrasions are, for me, the hardest things to watch. They are spontaneous and happen when you least expect it. Hon describes it as though someone throws acid in his eyes. I always feel so helpless, as there is nothing I can do except be there, keep him as comfortable as I can and to love him with all my heart while they heal.

We are very lucky; we have each other, and we battle EB together, we are a team. Hope and our love for each other keep us going. Hon's bravery and determination shine through every day. He is so unique. Hon is truly amazing in every way, he is my soul mate, my forever love and my extraordinarily brave butterfly.

> "AERODYNAMICALLY THE BUMBLEBEE SHOULDN'T BE ABLE TO FLY, BUT THE BUMBLEBEE DOESN'T KNOW THAT SO IT GOES ON FLYING ANYWAY."
>
> – Mary Kay Ash

Don't wrap us in cotton wool

By Wendy Hilling

"I can't let my skin win"

I was born with EB. I was kept in a cotton wool crib as a baby. We were known then as 'cotton wool babies'. I was protected and cushioned from life. I wasn't cuddled because it took my skin off. I spent months in hospital while they tried to sort out how to care for me. None of the doctors had ever seen EB.

My first memory of bandages is watching my mother ironing miles and miles of them. They would tumble off the ironing board and I would try to roll them up so they could be used again. They were scratchy and hard. They had to be tied on me.

I grew up wanting to do things and not being allowed to try. As soon as I left school I saved up for a pony. Yes, I got hurt, a lot at times. I had to work out how to ride and how to protect my skin as much as I could. It wasn't an easy journey. Skin sheared off from the inside of my legs and my hands got covered in blisters with each ride I went on. But I loved it. I could never walk far but I had freedom on my pony. I would ride alongside my friends with them on their bikes. I rode a lot without a saddle. I had to learn how to stay on my pony.

My mother told me years later that she dreaded a knock on the door to say I'd been badly hurt when I fell.

My parents took me to see a specialist in Guy's and St Thomas Hospital to tell him I was getting hurt horse riding; they thought I should stop.

His reply was, "she will stop when she gets hurt badly enough, let her try".

Years later we saw the same doctor. My Dad and my Mum said: "She didn't stop, she went on to get hurt over and over. She wouldn't stop."

He looked at me and said, "good for you".

When I met my now husband Peter, he tried to protect me. I knew we couldn't be together if he tried to clip my wings. Then I wrote this for him.

Let me get hurt

Let me get hurt, then you will see the mountains I can climb, the goals I can reach and the things I can do.

Let me get hurt so you can see what I can do and know the real me.

If you never let me try, how do I know how high I can climb and how far I have to fall, if indeed I ever have to fall at all.

Let me get hurt, otherwise my bandages bind my body - and my mind. I can't let my skin win.

Let me try.

So many children get stopped from doing things they long to do. We should be the judge of how much we are prepared to get hurt.

The pain is *our* pain.

"SHE MADE **BROKEN** LOOK **BEAUTIFUL** AND STRONG LOOK INVINCIBLE. SHE WALKED WITH THE UNIVERSE ON HER SHOULDERS AND MADE IT LOOK LIKE A PAIR OF WINGS."

– Ariana Dancu

EB builds empaths

By Chloe Mitchell

What is EB, I hear the world say

It's painful, unsightly, please don't let me catch it, they pray

They don't understand, they never were taught

These living angels have an unusual building block

Yes it's painful, incurable and it can be lethal too
but you cannot catch it, that is simply untrue

EB builds empaths, they understand struggle,
but they will embrace you with warmth and a cuddle

They know how it feels to have skin that tears,
feet that can't walk and touch that's too much to bare

Never will you meet kinder living beings

EB builds empaths, do you hear what I'm saying?

They would never wish another to feel their pain

yet others feel the need to be cruel, unwilling to learn, it's oh so vain

If you took but a minute to look it up,
you would see what warriors these angels are that you snub

Today choose kindness, don't be deterred

EB builds empaths, help us be heard

#FightEB

Butterfly girl

By Kairi Mitchell
(Age 5)

Talking about her blisters:

"Well, they are painful when you pop them

But Mummy gives me ice lollies and ice cream.

Having blisters is not fun

But you just have to take it

It's our skin condition that's doing it

We just can't control it

Some people have it too

I have it too

When you wear sandals sometimes blisters pop out of your skin

Sometimes your feet are in pain

It scares me when my Mummy has to lance my blisters on my feet

I don't like it when I need to pop my blisters

But I'm a butterfly girl; my feet don't stop me from flying"

"IF YOU STUMBLE, MAKE IT PART OF THE DANCE."

— Unknown

Dear diary...

By Naomi
(Age 10)

Today I got back from my year six residential. It was an awesome trip, and I was sad to leave. I had so much fun! And although my EB got in the way a little during some activities, I didn't let it stop me from having an amazing time.

We travelled to Tewkesbury on a coach, and thankfully I wasn't carsick for the journey (I have been carsick before, and it's horrible). We got there in time for an afternoon activity in separate groups. For my group it was canoeing, which lasted for a few hours on the river. My first big mistake. When you are on a canoe, you must use a paddle to move through the water. Moving that paddle through the water causes a lot of friction on your hands, as I found out. Of course, I still had a lot of fun, but by dinner that evening, I could already feel my fingers hurting, and the next day held more paddle-based fun. Fun for me, not my hand.

The next morning, we had kayaking and paddleboarding, both using paddles. I tried putting a dressing over my hands, but it soon came off and I had to do it without. By the end of the session, I was soaking wet and laughing with my friends, but then there was climbing after lunch. Thanks to my sore hands, I had to sit that one out. I was sad to miss out, but my friends still sat next to me when they weren't climbing, and I had fun that way instead. It wasn't all bad.

If I wanted to go to the toilet in the night, I had to go outside and along a path to get there. When you are tired and your feet are blistered and hurting, this is not nice. Somehow, my friends made it fun by taking me to the bathroom in my wheelchair instead, to save my feet. There was always an argument over who got to push me! Honestly, I don't get why it's so fun, but I was glad of the enthusiasm.

On Wednesday, we held a disco in the marquee. My feet were really hurting but I managed to ignore the pain and have fun anyway. In fact, the previous evening a friend taught me how to do the macarena in my wheelchair during the run-around quiz – a quiz where the answers were scattered around the site. The disco was probably my highlight of the week, and most of my classmates' as well. Yes, my feet hurt, but if you want to enjoy it, you must ignore that.

Throughout the week, my blisters created many painful obstacles, but thanks to everyone around me who supported and helped me, I still had one of the best weeks of my life.

When to wheelchair

By Carly

At the age of four, my daughter Naomi was, if I'm honest, already too big for the pushchair that we were using. We'd hung on to it like a safety net as people don't question or judge a child in a pushchair. They do question and judge a child in a wheelchair.

But she still needed something to get her from A to B. With EB Simplex, her feet – particularly in the summer months – are too blistered to let her walk any distance. So, we looked at our follow-on options.

Mentally, *I* was not ready for a wheelchair. I couldn't at that point accept that my daughter would need a wheelchair for life. Instead, we were prescribed an oversized pushchair, a Dobuggy. It did the job although it was cumbersome and stiff. We persevered with it for three years, really putting it through its paces in the very hilly area that we live in. It was on its last legs when we were finished with it.

Yet I was still not ready to accept the wheelchair. We investigated e-bikes and electric scooters. There was even a discussion about how we could fit a golf trolley battery to some home-fashioned transportation system. Thankfully, for Naomi at least, none of those came to fruition.

In fact, it was Naomi that made the decision: she wanted the wheelchair. "Mum," she said, "I'm too big for that pushchair so people stare anyway, and I want to be able to have control, not be pushed everywhere."

I had forgotten that Naomi would, as she got older, start to have her own plans for her mobility. I should have asked her sooner.

Our first wheelchair was a basic NHS-prescribed chair. It wasn't very exciting; it didn't have streamers or fancy wheels. But importantly, it was a self-propelled chair, giving Naomi the independence she wanted.

While she couldn't do much self-propelling because of her reduced muscle strength, and because too much would have led to blisters on her fingers, the option was there. This was a real milestone for me and at last the acceptance of the need for a wheelchair.

We've moved on from that chair to a rugged one, part funded by the NHS, which means we can go offroad and enjoy some wilder walks. Wherever we go, it goes. Even if it means that we push it empty for the day just in case Naomi needs it.

From a source of anxiety for me, the wheelchair has become a symbol of independence for Naomi and is now very much part of our EB family.

It's the Little Things!

By Bex Knight

For us a positive is we appreciate and celebrate the little things, that other people take for granted. The amount of love and joy they bring every day with a smile on their face, fighting another day just makes me so proud xx

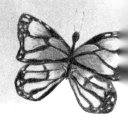

"YOU ARE *STRONG* WHEN YOU KNOW YOUR *WEAKNESSES.* YOU ARE BEAUTIFUL WHEN YOU APPRECIATE YOUR FLAWS. YOU ARE *WISE* WHEN YOU LEARN FROM YOUR *MISTAKES.*"

— Unknown

Eye of the Tiger

By Krystal Prescod

Q: If someone asked you "What is EB?", how would you answer? What's your first thought? This doesn't have to be the definition, but more what it is to you.

A: It's a very rare genetic skin condition that most people have never heard of. The main feature is fragile skin that easily blisters and shears; however, it affects everything!

To me, it is a challenge that I was given in life. I have had to learn how to take care of it and advocate for myself (with my Mum's help) before I ever had a diagnosis, and afterwards as there was no support for me growing up in Western Canada.

EB is something that helped me to learn problem solving at a young age. I didn't know about silicone dressings until my early 30s. I had to find the non-stick gauze pads and paper tape in the pharmacies. I had to learn how to ease the pain without the use of analgesics, such as massaging my feet gently with peppermint foot lotion, while avoiding all open wounds.

I have so much in life that I want to see, so I have had to learn about how to keep going despite the chronic pain of EB. The EB will always be there, but my opportunities to see or achieve the things I want in life may not be.

Q: What do you wish someone had told you about living with EB?

A: I wish someone told me about lancing blisters with hypodermic needles, as I used to have cuticle scissors for lancing blisters. The needle method has saved a significant amount of pain. I wish someone had told me about silicone dressings, as the drugstore methods caused additional skin trauma.

Q: What is a tip you would give to someone who has EB?

A: Tailor this life to your own unique EB needs. Find ways to have everything that is important to you, but your skin makes challenging. I always love seeing sparkly high heels, which obviously would be too painful with my EB. Instead, I have found some sparkly trainers and added insoles, and used preventative dressings until they are broken in. If you struggle to travel by normal methods, go on a cruise or look up disability travel tours. Our EB does not need to stop us from achieving things we want; it just might look a little different than originally thought.

Q: Which tip would you give to a parent/carer of a child, of any age, living with EB?

A: Have a positive atmosphere around dressing changes. Have your children lance their own blisters and change dressings as early as possible while supervising. When you go for a pedicure, it may be very ticklish but for you to do it yourself, it is not. Same thing applies to blisters: it may be very painful for your child to have someone else pop their blisters but for them to do it is much easier. My Mum started supervising and helping me take care of my own when I was six and it made both of our lives easier. My Mum was also happy when we did my blister care, which kept me happy and calm.

Q: Do you have a favourite quote(s) that you use in relation to your EB? Please do share and, if you would like to, please say why you like it.

A: "It is what it is". I like this because it strikes so true. It is what it is, I cannot change it. It is what it is, also seems to minimise the emotional impact.

Q: Anything else you would like to add? A fact about EB? A point of interest? Something you find fascinating?

A: For years, I struggled with chronic fatigue and aches and pains throughout my body, in addition to the EB. A family member recommended that I saw a naturopathic doctor. I wasn't getting anywhere with my GP as my blood tests were all in normal ranges, except for slightly elevated inflammatory markers, which were "dismissed" due to my EB. After a two-hour consultation, I was advised to stop eating gluten and dairy, and given a lot of great options of foods to eat. Within 36 hours I noticed huge improvements in my energy and no aches and pains. What I found fascinating was, as the inflammation decreased, so did a lot of my EB! Since having a more anti-inflammatory diet, my EB has dramatically improved. Less pain, less blisters!

Lastly, have fun with this life! Our EB lives may be a little different, but even in the lows we can bring fun and great memories. My Mum and I went to Las Vegas to celebrate my 25th birthday. This was before I realised that shoes with arch support were the worst ones for me, and I had some beautiful new trainers that were more breathable. Adding in all the walking of Las Vegas, and wearing the "wrong" shoes, I was unable to walk for the last two days. I couldn't even manage to get to the loo inside the hotel room.

My Mum went downstairs and rented me a mobilised scooter for the rest of our trip. Being 25 and not "looking" like I needed a mobilised scooter, I was crying at the thought of it. My Mum had said that I could either use it and enjoy the last two days or stay in the hotel room and miss out. So, after crying it out, and some kind and encouraging words from my Mum I was ready to go.

After having our breakfast, I was back to myself again and starting to have fun with it. Then I got a little cheeky, as we were on an overhead walkway, I told my Mum I needed to stop, I found the "Eye of the Tiger" song on my BlackBerry, and played it at full volume, then I sped by my Mum saying, "Come on Rocky!". I still to this day laugh when I think of it. I love little wins like that in life.

"SHE WAS POWERFUL NOT BECAUSE SHE WASN'T SCARED BUT BECAUSE SHE WENT ON SO STRONGLY, DESPITE THE FEAR."

— Atticus

Endless Battle

By Melinda Venczel
(Age 42)

I live with EB, Kindler Syndrome. I'm from Romania and have been in UK since 2011, living in Cardiff at the moment. I am the luckiest person as I'm in the care of a great team at Guy's and St Thomas Hospital in London. I've written this poem about my life with EB.

I dare to dream, I dare to love
My fragile skin's the one I'm scared
I let my soul to speak for me
I let my eyes to tell you more

I'm grateful for your care and love
When I'm in pain and can't do more
I'll fight again after I rest
As this is what I can do best

Don't love me for the way I look
Don't judge me for the steps I took
It is my way of showing how
I do my best and dream high

"WHEN YOU HAVE A RARE DISEASE, YOU FACE TWO BATTLES. ONE BEING THE ILLNESS ITSELF, AND THE OTHER, LIVING IN A WORLD WHERE SO FEW PEOPLE UNDERSTAND WHAT YOU'RE UP AGAINST."

— *Anon*

The miracle and complexity of an EB baby

By Filipa and William Hinton

Mum:
As I sit scrolling through my phone, I find my birth video, and fondly recall the day that Arthur and Finlay were born. My husband, Will, was wearing a GoPro camera on his head in the delivery room so that I could later relive the moment they came into our lives, as lying down on a table in theatre for my C-section meant I could not see what he could see. I wanted to relish that moment for years to come.

There is this one moment in the video I press pause that stands out. This is the moment that Arthur was born, and the doctors held him up like a scene from The Lion King; they tell us that baby one is here.

Looking at this video now, I can see the doctors both staring intently at his feet. In this moment frozen in time, they knew something was wrong with one of our twins.

The kind nurse sitting by my side tells me quietly that Arthur has been born with some damage to his feet, but she calmly tells me that it sometimes happens with birth trauma, and not to worry. I am too excited to hear her attentively as a few minutes later baby two is here, Finlay, born still inside an intact amniotic sac. This, we are told, is quite a rare event.

This is a happy day, both boys are here and healthy, or so I thought. But from one rare event in Finlay's birth, we would soon find out we have a rare disease that would be with Arthur for life.

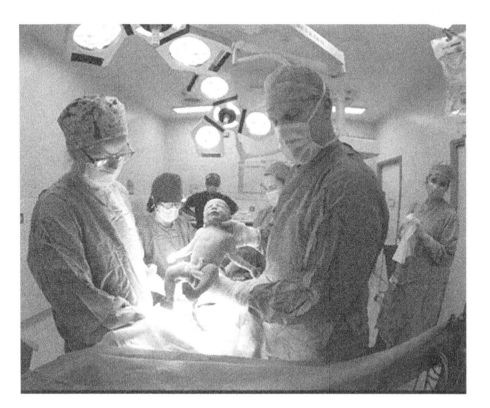

Dad:
I tried to be a calm presence for Filipa as she went through this major operation. When Arthur was born, the midwife told me the same information that Filipa describes about the missing skin from his feet: "Sometimes this can happen" and "not to worry". With those reassuring words, I did not feel concerned. And, I barely had a moment to process this news with Finlay arriving just a few moments later.

With a lack of cots available on the ward on a particularly busy day for babies being born, I was lucky enough to stay at the hospital beyond the two hours after delivery (as per restrictions in place during the Covid-19 pandemic), through to midnight, to hold my sons for the first time, and do my best to help Filipa. What a day it had been! So much excitement and so much to process… and with that I drive back home.

Mum:
It wasn't until day three that a dermatologist that works in a building across the car park sent a photographer to the ward to take some photos of Arthur's damaged skin. By this time his feet had not been tended to, and every time I ask a nurse on the ward, "what shall I do with his feet?", they say to just leave them until we hear from the doctors.

Within hours of those photos being taken, the dermatologist is at my bed telling me she thinks it is a condition called Epidermolysis Bullosa, and she would be sending a referral immediately to Great Ormond Street Hospital (GOSH). I am taken back as I have never heard of this condition and did not know what it meant for my three-day-old child. She just tells me to not Google it and we will wait to hear from GOSH for next steps. At this point, I am completely overwhelmed having been in hospital by myself as a first-time Mum to twins who don't seem to ever sleep or eat at the same time. And the Covid-19 restrictions mean that I cannot get any help from the outside world. Unfortunately, the staff on the ward are so busy that they cannot provide help either. I breakdown, cry, and call my husband to tell him the news.

Dad:
Filipa phoned me, clearly upset with news about Arthur. Like her, I had never heard the words, Epidermolysis Bullosa or EB. Although, Filipa said she had been advised not to Google it, I could not stop myself from doing so. I didn't know what to think, but just focused on trying to give my wife positive thoughts. "You're in the best place... the doctors will know what to do... you will be home soon."

Mum:
It's day four of becoming a Mum, I am confused and overwhelmed but I keep focusing on my boys. A nurse comes to see me in the morning and tells me GOSH have sent some communication. They tell me there are specific instructions on how to handle the baby and how to carefully change nappies to avoid further damage. But they don't have a printer at hand, so they will be coming to see me later with this information. They also mention that GOSH are visiting tomorrow so they will be moving me from a multiple person ward to a private room, and that my husband will be allowed to join briefly for the consultation. I look forward to having the support from my husband but dreading what this means... an entire team coming from London to see me.

The hours go past, and no-one comes and shows me this document. At 10pm I call a nurse and cry and say, 'what's going on, why is no one giving me information, or helping me understand how to better care for my son?' She calls her ward manager who comes and sits with me, and finally shows me the document they managed to print earlier in the day. They had been reluctant to show it to me without explaining why. But the nurse finally took a few minutes to sit and read through it with me, showing me what the document means. For example, they demonstrate how to roll over the baby with open hands to minimise pressure points and friction when changing a nappy. She also tells me that I should use a specific aerosol spray called Emollin to clean his bottom, but it's stuck in health and safety bureaucracy as it was considered to be highly flammable, and in their opinion not safe to be used in the ward (according to the pharmacy).

I struggle to understand why I should not have access to this medicine now if it means helping my son. I am in disbelief but too tired to fight her over this. In the meantime, I am completely unaware that with every stroke with cotton soaked in water, I am causing further damage to my son's nappy area. The next day he was blistered all over that area now too.

On day five, we finally get to meet the EB team, three lovely health care professionals come to see us, speak to us for an hour, take our boy to a separate room to take a skin sample, and we each go to another room for blood samples. They kindly explained the condition and what it could mean if it's confirmed that he has EB. They let us absorb the information and then show us how to lance his blisters and to wrap the damaged areas with dressings they came armed with.

And just like that, our journey into EB starts, and the long daily wound dressing sessions.

Dad:
I visit the hospital in Filipa's private room, and I am greeted by a team of three friendly faces from the EB team at GOSH, and of course, to my relief, my very tired and emotional wife. There was so much information to process, covering what EB is and the different types and the need for regular wound care sessions.

The nurses demonstrate how to lance Arthur's blisters and apply his dressings... we don't know if we can do this. However, it is clear that we do not have a choice.

We are told that tomorrow we need to demonstrate to a nurse that we can lance and drain Arthur's blisters and change his dressings before Filipa and the boys can be discharged from hospital. We are lucky that with all this new and daunting information, the ward manager allows me to stay the night at the hospital to help Filipa throughout the night.

Despite having much anxiety and fear, we successfully show the nurse that we can perform the various tasks for Arthur's wound care, and we go home later that day as first-time parents and as carers.

In our meeting with the EB team (and later on, with various healthcare professionals), we were told that as Arthur's parents, we are "the experts" for managing his EB. While this is true, in the first few days/weeks of his life, hearing those words felt terrifying, particularly as we had no prior knowledge about EB before his birth. What did this mean? We know nothing about EB; does it mean they know nothing too? It's an incredibly confusing and overwhelming thought.

In hindsight, I believe these words are said to parents to make them feel empowered when caring for their children that have EB. For example, we now know not to put any type of plaster on Arthur's skin (due to blistering around the edges) or particular creams/gels, despite an EB specialist saying those work well for other EB patients.

Mum:
The first few weeks were filled with the excitement of being a parent for the first time, the love I feel for my twins and my husband, but also this cloud of sadness that my son is in constant pain. All I want to do is hold him and tell him I wish I could take it away. The EB team kept in touch and would come visit in person from time to time. These visits are an invaluable support that I will forever be grateful for.

I remember this moment vividly. I was sat at a makeshift treatment table in our living room, we made do with my old office desk and a baby mat, doing Arthur's wound care while the EB nurse observed. I start to cry and tell her, "I feel like I am being a nurse... all I want is to be a Mum right now!" This feeling has never gone away completely but has definitely eased over time.

For one day per week, I am able to just be a Mum because we receive support from the amazing children's community nursing team that help with Arthur's wound care, allowing us to just be parents. This was something the EB nurses organised to take the emotional and physical burden off us as Arthur's carers.

For the first few months, I spend all waking hours of the day browsing the internet and all literature about EB. "Can I really do this?" I keep questioning myself and thinking, "will it always feel like this?" I eventually come across a few EB Facebook groups, "the butterfly skin charity", Debra, and connect with these groups. These have become a real lifeline to us as a family; the doctors and nurses can only help so much. These communities have many of the answers I have been looking for, and at any hour of the day. But most importantly, they listen and understand our problems, something we have struggled to communicate to those closest to us.

Despite how hard living with EB is and seeing our child go through all he does, our little warrior keeps us going, and his incredible ability to keep smiling is all that matters right now. With his determination, the EB community support, and some special people we have met along the way, we have figured out how to do the basics in looking after our son. These include how to safely bathe him with soft cushioning in the bath, foods he can have, surfaces he should sleep and sit on, turning clothes inside out to limit damage to his skin against the seams, finding shoes that are soft but provide enough support for his ankles as he learns to walk... the list is endless. We chose to live day by day to keep things as simple as possible.

The following photo shows the very first time I braved putting Arthur tummy down at four months old, to work on his neck strength. Until that day, I feared causing damage on his tummy, an area that has never blistered before, and I wanted so desperately to keep it that way. I have the message fixed in my head from the health care professionals, do not handle him too much to avoid further damaging his skin. However, the Facebook family reminded me that he needed to develop and work his neck strength too. They reminded me, he heals too. They kindly suggested the correct type of pillow to use and to make sure to position a sheepskin under him to minimise friction, and I did it. In the back of my mind, I kept thinking, "how badly will the damage be when we look at his chest later this evening during wound care?" His big smile was everything. He was so happy that he was finally seeing the world from a different direction!

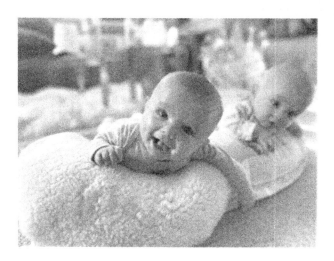

Dad:

As for any parents to newborns, the first few weeks were a huge adjustment, with many restless nights for feeding and nappy changes, and of course the dreaded, colic! But with Arthur, we constantly worried about how we moved him (he constantly lay on his back on a sheepskin rug), and the pain that he was in. I remember calling 111 late in the evening to request a prescription for paracetamol, to know the dose required at such a young age (the bottles don't list this for younger than 3 months), and driving to the pharmacy late at night, desperate to relieve my son's pain.

I also remember that the clamp on Arthur's umbilical cord was removed at the hospital, under the EB team's advice, as there was concern that this may rub his skin and cause further damage. It took two to three weeks to eventually dry and fall off, but as he had a lot of redness and inflammation on his tummy, we sought medical advice and we were advised to take him to hospital. He was treated with antibiotics for a possible infection and admitted overnight, as they had never seen a patient with EB and wanted to treat it to be on the safe side. However, his blood test results eventually came back and showed that he did not have an infection... this appeared to just be a side of EB we were not aware of. It eventually healed on its own in the days following Arthur's discharge from hospital. This was the first of many antibiotic treatments Arthur has had since he was born, often to err on side of caution, when his wounds seem infected and the skin swabs take 3-4 days to come back with the results.

From speaking to other parents, this seems to be a common problem with EB. One parent asked if we had considered prophylactic antibiotics to keep his infections at bay, as she did with her son. She showed us all the supporting evidence that continued use of antibiotics (at low dose) is less likely to lead to antibiotic resistance than stronger doses in response to new infections. After running this suggestion by the EB consultant, they agreed this was a good way forward. This was a game changer for our son.

We also had a lot of difficulty getting Arthur to feed initially. Our sons were bottle fed, but the teat of the bottle caused a lot of damage to Arthur's lips and gums, which left him in a lot of pain and refusing his bottle. This was very worrying for us as we feared that Arthur would need to go back into hospital until he could feed properly again. Thankfully, the EB team introduced us to the Haberman bottle. This was ideal for him as it provides a steady stream of milk, which required less suction than a normal bottle. After a few days, he had taken back to regular feeding and the damage that the previous bottle caused, soon healed. Another obstacle overcome.

Mum:
I remember the joy it gave us seeing Finlay, jumping up and down on the Jumperoo and how Arthur would giggle looking at him doing it. Inside I thought, "why can't I be brave and put Arthur in the Jumperoo too?" But I knew the guidance was not to hold your child under their armpits so, how will I get him in and out? I debated this for far too many months until I finally decided to be creative and come up with a makeshift pulley system with one of his silk sheets. He was ecstatic to finally be given the chance to do it. He had the biggest smile and inside I felt so guilty that I kept letting my fear hold him back from such moments.

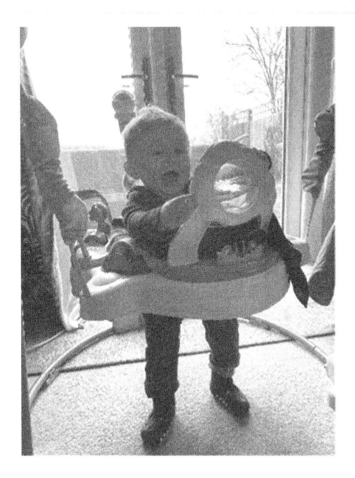

Mum & Dad:
Day by day, we manoeuvred through life with managing our son's EB. We did most things, one hurdle at a time. From safe travelling in a car, working out how to minimise damage to his neck by finding a car seat that does not use neck straps; to flying to Portugal to visit family and give Mum the opportunity to meet her grandchildren before she passed away. We took him swimming to a local pool after a long time, giving into our fears of thinking it is impossible with all his dressings and wounds, while our other twin fully enjoyed this activity.

Another big hurdle was considering whether to give up my job to stay home to look after my son. This would mean financially we could no longer afford to live in our house or put Finlay in nursery too. But with the encouragement and support from Debra, the children's community nursing team, and the EB community, we found the most fantastic nursery that met Arthur's needs and was not afraid of the challenge. Arthur's cheeky personality really came out by attending nursery with his twin brother. For us, this sense of normality is important, and we can see in his little face how important being able to do things other kids do makes him happy. This was the confirmation we did the right thing for him despite all our reservations. We decided on that day that we would try to never hold him back, and to do our utmost to figure out a way to help him achieve his goals.

We are two years into this journey and although we feel we have gotten into a routine, it is only very slowly getting easier. However, Arthur is showing us how to "thrive with EB", a quote we often hear from the *MiaThrives* podcasts, which we aim to live by.

"DEFINITION OF A HERO:
A CHILD OR ADULT WITH EB WHO
WAKES UP EVERY MORNING
READY TO TRY AGAIN."

– Unknown

The EB armour

By Hannah West

It would seem that the lack of protection EB gives your skin results in the formation of emotional armour and the willingness to fight. Not just for the person living with the condition (and crikey they are some of the toughest, most inspirational people I have met), but for the whole family.

There are so many battles you face, each leaving you more scarred, yet tougher. As parents, our first was diagnosis. Three years of not understanding what caused the mysterious blisters that made our daughter scream. Three years of never knowing why any fun play time would end in cut knees and tears no matter how gentle the knock or tumble while others just got up unscathed and carried on. Three years of being told we were imagining things and there wasn't a problem. And when we finally found a locum who listened, being told by a partner in our GP practice that hospital appointments were expensive to the NHS and we should have second thoughts about taking our daughter for one when we didn't need it.

The relief of finally being listened to showed us we were right to fight. And so, for the next battle we were tougher. This was the start of the formation of our armour – the chainmail if you like. Our child had EB. She needed us.

Holding her down to do her blisters while she cried, and I cried because I couldn't just make everything better for her while my Mum cried for us both because she couldn't help her baby either. But then she needed us to be strong. So, the armour formed. And Mum and I cried our tears away from her; sharing our sadness at the injustice of it all and the guilt and the worry so we became each other's armour.

And then there are the words that can find a chink in the armour. Doctors making you feel like inept parents. Hurtful comments from people who don't understand. And sometimes from others who do. Why are you going on again? It's not that bad. My child has it worse. But then others sweep in. Parents of children who deal with far more. Who let you know that it's ok to feel as you do. It is unfair. You're allowed to be sad. And hurt. Who are a complete inspiration. Who share stories and support. And so you know that you can do this. It makes your armour stronger. And you learn that it's important to take the armour off sometimes and share the emotional wounds to help them heal.

And so, we all wear our armour, surrounding her with support and love – her cavalry. From aunties who literally run marathons to sisters who may be extremely annoying but who will also stand up to any stranger to deal with undesired comments and questions. From family members who've grown in love and understanding to friends who show support and kindness way beyond their years.

Armour may be heavy and uncomfortable. And it doesn't shield you from getting things wrong and endless parental guilt. But to protect this wonderful, inspirational, caring, infuriating, beautiful person, as parents we will buckle ourselves in every day to face whatever battle is next.

Love

By Rachel Lee-Davis

For me there are so many positives. I feel like I have a 2nd family in the EB community, everyone just gets it. I love sharing EB posts, then see a wave of them going out across friends, especially EB friends bringing awareness to outside world.

As much as bath and dressing changes take hours and hours daily, I love that I get to spend this time with Hon.

When Covid hit I worked from home due to needing to sheild hubbie again I am grateful for the 24/7 time I am home and now able to spend quality time together Hons EB is so bad now, but we enjoy making the most of every moment, just chilling out watching movies together.

I love when we meet people who have never heard of EB, especially in medical profession, Hon is world's first with EB to have a kidney transplant, he really is pioneering, people are inspired and for me I am so proud of my hubbie every day!

We have wonderful friends through the EB community that I know are lifelong friends.

The Corneal Abrasions are the worst, but I am here and just snuggle up while we let them heal in the dark together.

Probably the biggest positive for me, is that EB enabled me to meet my soulmate, my forever love. I was a district nurse when I first met Hon. After our care was finished we remained good friends and the rest is history. XXX

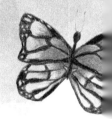

> "I THOUGHT I WOULD HAVE TO TEACH MY CHILD ABOUT THE WORLD. IT TURNS OUT I HAVE TO TEACH THE WORLD ABOUT MY CHILD"
>
> – Unknown

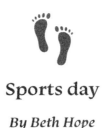

Sports day

By Beth Hope

Sports day is filled with fun, friendly competiveness and a great day for parents and children... for those without a disability.

The night before: "Make sure you wear two pairs of socks tomorrow to help pad your feet, how are your feet?" I ask.

"They're a little blistered, but I should be okay tomorrow " Isaac replies.

On the day, all the parents arrive onto the Sports Day field and my first thought is, 'wow, I hadn't realised how large this field is'. All the activities are spread around this huge field and my mind is overthinking how Isaac is going to manage walking from each event, never mind doing all of the activities as well. I spot Isaac sitting amongst his class peers. A huge grin meets me as he spots me in the crowd of parents. I grin back and feel happy to be here on this sunny day.

All of the parents walk around with their child's class watching the activities.

The first event is a lateral barrier jump. What happened to egg and spoon races?! The aim is to keep your legs closed together over and jump over a hurdle side to side and someone stands in front of you counting how many jumps you can do in one minute. I'm standing close to where Isaac is sitting and I see the panic on his face. He looks at me and says: "I don't think I'll be able to do that, my feet are already sore from walking today."

"Don't worry," I say, "do whatever events you can and just sit this one out."

Isaac's teaching assistant comes over to me and explains Isaac can only do the throwing ones if he wants to. Isaac agrees to this and feels a bit more relieved. As we walk away from this event another child is crying because he only did 38 jumps compared with his friend who did 46. Isaac pulls a face; I know he is wishing he could have done that one without the embarrassment of being able to do just one jump in front of his class mates and the fact that just one would have caused him a lot of pain.

Isaac performs in the throwing events and continues to walk around the field in his class. I kick myself for not bringing his wheelchair so that he can have a bit more comfort in going to each activity. I thought he would be okay because it's only on the school field, he isn't going very far, but it is the amount of walking to and from activities, standing, sitting, and even the friction from moving his feet in the throwing events. They all make an impact on his skin.

An hour and 30 minutes into the event. Isaac is on the brink of tears. He comes over to me, emotion bubbling over, and says: "I want to go home, my feet are so sore. I can't do the events, there's so many more to go, and we're only halfway through."

We walk over to his teacher and explain that Isaac really needs to stop what he's doing. Isaac also has Tourette's and when he's stressed or in a lot of pain from his EB, his Tourette's gets more severe.

The teacher doesn't want Isaac to leave. He explains that cheering on other students will be really fun for him and supportive to the other students.

As we walk back Isaac gets very upset. I take him away from the group and we sit down in the shade.

"I just want to be a normal kid," Isaac cries. "I want to be able to run and do everything like a normal kid."

"I know, I know" I try to soothe. "EB sucks."

After 15 minutes of sitting out, the teacher comes over to us and asks why Isaac isn't supporting the other students by cheering them on. I explain that Isaac was feeling upset that he couldn't join in, and he was experiencing a lot of pain.

"Can you not take some painkillers?" he asked.

"He's already taken his max dosage this morning. He still has a couple of hours to go before he can take anymore."

Having dealt with many people doubting me and my blisters over my lifetime, I can see that the teacher is wondering what the big fuss is. He's a new teacher who hasn't seen Isaac's skin before. He is young and even though he's a good teacher, you can tell he has not come across many children with disabilities before.

After a discussion about going home to get Isaac's wheelchair, the teacher says that they have one on site and offers to go and get it to relieve Isaac from standing.

While he goes into get it, I say to Isaac, "quick, take off your shoes and socks!"

Isaac is puzzled and I explain that the only way your teacher is going to understand is if he sees your feet right now. To suggest this I have to overcome my own memories from when I was a teenager, when a PE teacher told me to show him my blisters. I was so angry at the time as I had a lot of blisters underneath the skin and I couldn't even show him to prove how horrible he was being by not believing me.

In this situation, it felt different. There was a need to explain and sometimes the severity of the blistering is all you need to show for an explanation.

The teacher returns with a wheelchair and kneels beside Isaac. He looks down at his bare feet. There is a look of understanding, and an empathy develops. The teacher isn't a bad person, there is just a lack of education and here, we are educating him.

Isaac's feet look quite messy, there are cut blisters that we've previously treated and are healing. There is old skin coming off where old blisters have been, and making way for new skin underneath and then there are all the new blisters. The various sized liquid filled bubbles dotted around his toes, ankles and insides of the soles where his shoes plimsolls have rubbed the most and exposed him to new blisters.

In this moment, I know that Isaac will never be doubted by this particular teacher again. As for the future, I know we will continue the struggle for this disability to be seen. We will have to fight for recognition, understanding and empathy in every remaining school year we have left for Isaac, as that was what happened for me and my father and my grandmother. The generational cycles of fighting to be treated fairly with our disability. I hope with more awareness and education that this fight doesn't have to continue for Isaac and his children.

> "I DON'T LIVE WITH EB;
> EB LIVES WITH ME."
>
> — *Unknown*

Oscar

By Jake Fish
(Dad to Oscar, age four)

My name is Oscar and I'm only four,

I've got a condition which leaves me quite sore.

It's called EB which makes my layers fragile and thin.

They say it's like having butterfly skin.

But even when my feet can't handle no more

I find a way to cross the floor.

Because I'm a brave boy who everyone adores.

Mummy and Daddy help me a lot
they have to pop the blisters or they just wouldn't stop.

Plasters, bandages and cream, all that I need to keep my skin clean.

"SOME PEOPLE NEVER MEET THEIR HERO. I GAVE BIRTH TO MINE."

— Unknown

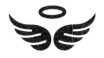

An EB angel

By Jo Connelly

When Lewis was born, we noticed straight away that something was wrong. His feet and wrists looked raw and sore. He was quickly taken away to intensive care and treated for sepsis, but no one could tell us what was wrong. It was horrifying!

The next day the consultant dermatologist came and said that although he had never seen a case in real life, he thought Lewis had Epidermolysis Bullosa. We couldn't even pronounce it let alone understand it.

Over the next couple of days, we started to Google it and what we saw left us in terror. What would this mean for our baby? How could we watch our child cope with so much pain?

Then the specialist EB nurses came from Birmingham Children's Hospital. Angels who showed us how best to care for our wee boy. While they were there, we noticed a young girl was watching everything they did. The next day one of the neonatal intensive care unit (NICU) nurses - another angel - asked if we had noticed the young girl watching Lewis. She explained that she was on work experience in the NICU. They had never had anyone on school work experience before but this girl was keen to be a nurse. And here is the bit that gives me goosebumps every time I tell anyone. She wanted to speak to us because she had EB! She had never met anyone outside her family with EB and that is why she had been watching Lewis so closely.

We of course agreed to speak to her, and she explained how EB affected her and how she could still do most things she wanted to.

I cannot begin to express the hope that gave to us as parents in that dark and terrifying time and I sometimes wonder if she was actually a real person.

Those first few weeks of Lewis' life are a blur but I'm sure her name was Georgia. So Georgia, if you read this, thank you for being in the right place at the right time and for bringing hope when we needed it the most.

"WHEN I FIRST HEARD ABOUT EB, IT WAS QUITE HARD TO GRASP THE INTENSITY OF THE CONDITION. IT'S ABOUT THE MOST INSANE SKIN DISORDER YOU CAN IMAGINE. NOT EVEN THE BEST PSORIASIS CREAM CAN HELP. AND WHEN YOU REALISE IT ALSO AFFECTS THE INTERNAL ORGANS, THEN YOU SEE IT AS DIABOLICAL."

— Eddie Vedder

EB

By Amelia West
(Age 10)

EB is a terrible skin condition
It can cause a lot of pain
People have tried to find a cure
But all their efforts are in vain

It can happen to anyone
And sometimes removes skin
It can cause blistering
And can be upsetting to their kin

But there's a charity called Debra
Who fight EB
They have a logo with a butterfly not a zebra

My sister has EB
She normally isn't that nice
But whatever she does she is skating on thin ice

Life is very hard for her
But she continues day to day
With a normal routine
In a normal way

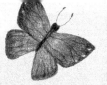

We celebrate a bruise!

Tracey O'Donnell

It makes me value the things I do in between the blisters. The adventures before the pain are often worth the pain, I make sure I fill the good days with as much as I can so I remember the good and not the blisters. I have also lost a few friends along the way who didn't like having to limit themselves to 'my pace' so I now only have true friends, those who don't care how much I limit them as they are happy to do what I can with me. XX

Lucy Shaw

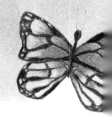

> *"EB: THE WORST CONDITION YOU HAVE NEVER HEARD OF."*
>
> — Unknown

Learning from a mutation

By Jo Linton

When our daughter Poppy was born everything was perfect, or so we thought. We were overjoyed that she had arrived safely after a week of being induced. We came home on the Sunday and we started to get in to our new role of first time parents.

The midwife came to check her on day two and noticed that her cord had a little blister on it. She thought no more of it. On day five, heel prick day we had noticed that her cord blister was getting slightly bigger. The midwife did her heel prick again and then we noticed she got a blister there - we now know it's because it was a trauma point.

By the next Sunday the blister on her heel was almost as big as a golf ball. As most people know, you don't burst blisters, so we left it alone. But then it burst, and Poppy turned really pale. We took her the local Accident & Emergency, but they couldn't tell us what was wrong, so we were shipped off to the city hospital.

Poppy was just eight days old. We had noticed by now that tiny little blisters had appeared on other parts of her body. The doctors didn't know what was wrong. It wasn't until a dermatologist came to see her that Epidermolysis Bullosa was mentioned, although he had never met anyone with it. We went onto Google, trying to find out about the condition and I can honestly say I've never been as scared in my life from what I saw.

They called the team from Birmingham Children's Hospital who took a look at her and confirmed that it was EB. They took her off to have a skin shave to confirm which version of Epidermolysis Bullosa she had, showed us how to dress her blisters, showed us how to lance her blisters and generally how to care for her. We were told to only hold our 11-day-old baby on a silk pillow, and to put her clothes inside out to avoid the seams rubbing her. I remember when the team left, we just broke down in tears. I was so sad for my baby having to go through life with all this pain. But we said we wouldn't wrap her in cotton wool and would let her live life to the max. If something didn't work we would change things.

We got the results that she had a brand-new mutation: Epidermolysis Bullosa Generalised Severe.

Now, she is almost six years old and has started to lance her blisters herself. She is such a happy little girl and the bravest person I know.

"IT TAKES UNIMAGINABLE STRENGTH TO CONTINUALLY ENDURE, PERSIST AND OVERCOME. PEOPLE WITH EB AREN'T WEAK. THEY'RE THE STRONGEST HUMAN BEINGS YOU'LL EVER MEET"

— Unknown

As fragile as a butterfly

By Clair Charij, for my son Brad

My baby boy was born in September 1999.

Nine pounds, 1 ounce and I was told he was fine.
My Bradley was here and I am now a Mum.
Then the midwife noticed a blister on his thumb.
"It must just be from sucking his thumb in the womb."
These were the words said in the delivery room.

A few weeks old, a blood blister on his toe.
The health visitor assistant blamed the babygro.
"Has your Mummy squeezed your little feet in too tight?"
I felt such a bad Mum, but what she said was not right.

A week later, another huge blister we found,
On his ankle, size of tenpence and perfectly round.
I took Brad to the doctors to get these wounds checked out,
But the GP tutted and said, "you've nowt to worry about."

Mummy instincts took over, I just knew that something was wrong.
The GP thought I was going crazy, but my feelings were so strong.
We changed doctor's surgery, and sought real care for our son.
And remain forever grateful for everything they have done.

The new GP had his suspicions and my God, he was right.
So then referred to Swindon Hospital, with a diagnosis in sight.
The consultant we saw in dermatology was an expert indeed.
Being helpful and friendly, she certainly did succeed.

But the diagnosis she thought it was, she'd only seen once before,
With one other patient, who was covered in blisters so sore.
So, this consultant warned us not to Google the diagnosis EB,
because the horrific information would be heart-breaking to see.

So of course, I was terrified but I wanted and needed to know.

And the different types of EB on the Internet terrified us so.
Infection, cancer, death and a life full of pain,
With medication, and dressings and nothing to gain.

January 2000, we were referred to Great Ormond Street,
For the EB Specialist team to examine Brad's feet.
Lots of questions, many photos and we were so sad.
We were so vulnerable then, so we went to London with Dad.
They asked if we were related, as what Brad had was so rare?
As awkward as the question was, the specialists really did care.

Recessive Dystrophic EB was the name.
All I looked for was answers and who was to blame?
Was this my fault for having shingles in pregnancy?
Or for stopping the breastfeeding so suddenly?

Although they tried to reassure us that Brad will be okay.
I knew this was lifelong, and Brad could suffer every day.
The things we take for granted; all the normal things we do;
Eating, drinking, sleeping, walking and even going to the loo.
All these routine things in life; our Brad endured so much.
We had to lance every blister and we were frightened to touch.

The EB Nurses were angels, always at the end of the phone.
But we had to teach our local doctors and nurses at home.
As what we were going through, they had never seen before.
The different dressings, lotions, medicine and so much more.

Sharing our experience because Brad's EB was so unique,
Though we knew by now, it was mild and the future was not bleak.

2023 and Brad deals with the EB in his own way.
Happy and settled with his girlfriend and lives for every day.
He still has the check-ups at St. Thomas' every year.
And shares anything he needs to; with the ones he holds so dear.

But it still remains so sad, to see all Brad has to endure.
Which is why we give to Debra and hope they'll soon find a cure.

To raise awareness of EB, I have a Debra butterfly tattoo.
On my left hand, very visible and the butterfly is blue.
When people ask what it means and they question me why?
I tell them that EB skin is, 'As fragile as a butterfly'.

"COURAGE DOESN'T ALWAYS ROAR. SOMETIMES COURAGE IS THE LITTLE VOICE AT THE END OF THE DAY THAT SAYS I'LL TRY AGAIN TOMORROW."

– Mary Anne Radmacher

Living with EB

By Vie Portland

Imagine how it feels to have a stone in your shoe. It's uncomfortable. It can make you walk awkwardly. And then you can take off your shoe, remove the stone, and go back to your normal.

We can't.

When I'm asked to describe what EB is to me, I say that, on a good day, it feels like my shoes are filled with stones, but, the thing is, I'm not wearing shoes; this is my skin.

On a bad day, I say it feels like my skin has been torn open with a rusty razor blade, flaming lava put underneath, and then my skin is sewn up again with a blunt needle.

Walking on blistered feet doesn't mean just your feet hurt; your whole gait is out of balance, causing further discomfort, more pain, in joints, in backs.

When you get an itch, don't you love a good scratch? When you hit that sweet spot, it feels so good to stop the itch. How often do you need to do this?

For me - for many of us with EB - we itch all of the time. Sometimes, it's like a low hum; you can feel it, you know it's there, but, mostly, you can ignore it.

Then, there are the times when I itch so much that I fantasise about tearing my skin off and rubbing it on a cheese grater or rubbing against my cats' giant scratching posts.

But I can't. That would cause more damage to my skin.

A blister in the throat can feel like being stabbed with a sharpened chopstick.

Our skin can feel so hot. Not hot as in a lovely sunny day hot, but hot as in being in a scalding hot bath. Our skin can feel like fire. Imagine when you get bad sunburn, the heat, the stinging - that's frequently our skin.

Yet, we have to wear more layers. Layers to protect our skin from rubbing against other bits of skin. Layers to protect us from the damage of other clothes. Layers to hold dressings in place. Layers to protect us from external damage.

EB is a cruel, ironic, disability. For many of us, heat is a trigger, yet we need to wear more clothes. Many of us have very low Vitamin D levels, yet it can hurt to sit in the sun.

Many of us in the community have had someone, many someone's, say, "but it's just a blister; I get blisters when I wear new shoes, too." But our blisters are different. Our blisters can become huge. Not huge as in the size of a 2p piece, but huge as in engulfing toes, heels, fingers, arms …

It's easy to forget how important skin is. We think to protect our hearts, our lungs, our other internal organs, but we forgot that our skin is the largest organ, covering us inside and out.

For those of us with EB, we can never forget.

It's not all Bad

By Vie Portland

I have joked frequently since my diagnosis that I am medically exempt from ironing and vacuuming. Ironing because of the heat and friction on my hands, and vacuuming because of a couple of the other chronic pain conditions I have that were caused by having undiagnosed EB for so long. I'm very happy that I can skip out on housework!

I mention in my story that I am very grateful for the EB community, in the UK and globally. I have learned from them, laughed with them, and love them. There are people in my life, that I would hate to be without, that wouldn't be in my life if it weren't for EB.

I have had opportunities come my way that wouldn't have happened if I didn't have EB. The first public talk I gave was for Debra UK; I had no confidence then, and didn't believe anyone would find anything I had to say interesting, but that was the start of me believing that I am the expert, as all of us that live with disabilities are, in my conditions, and that people are interested in learning. Now, public speaking is something I love doing, whether that be about EB, about hidden disabilities, or about other aspects of my story and my work.

I have attended fancy dinners, balls, and posh events through the charity so I could schmooze with people that don't know about EB.

I have had incredible weekends away with other people with EB, again through Debra UK. To spend time with other people who understand why so many of us eat slowly; why some cutlery is awful to use; why we leap over those bobbly bits at crossings even though we're hobbling before and after; how simply existing at times can be exhausting yet we still carry on if there's something that's important to do or that brings joy; who laugh at the silly, or dark, jokes about the condition; who bemoan about particular clothing and shoes; all of these things and far more are the reasons why these weekends are invaluable, and something that many of us start looking forward to as soon as we're heading home from one.

Having EB has contributed to me being the person I am. It's made me realise how important it is to believe someone who says that something makes their disability or condition worse because I know there are things that many people wouldn't understand about EB. It's made me realise how important it is to have physical affection with those we love and trust when, so often, it can feel like we are just a medical specimen to be prodded and poked.

And having EB has made me realise how incredible I am, how incredible all of us that live with the condition are, for getting up and carrying on, and finding the best way to live our lives, despite the constant pain and discomfort. We're all bloody marvelous!

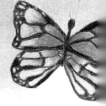

Acknowledgements

The first thanks must go to every person that has contributed to making this book happen: the writers and the poets for sharing their stories, even though, in many cases, it was hard for them to do so; to the two young people who created the beautiful cover design, Naomi Fields and Charlotte West; and to the two people who edited, formatted, and made this book something you could hold in your hands (or on your device), Carly Fields and Mark Clubb. You are all brilliant! Thank you to all of you for taking another of my big ideas and making it a reality. I appreciate you all so much.

Two charities are mentioned frequently in the book: Debra UK and Cure EB. The charities have helped many of us for several different reasons, from practical living advice, to benefits guidance, to grants, to research, to making events happen where lots of us can meet in person. We are all very grateful for you.

Thank you to our EB medical teams based in Great Ormond Street Hospital and St. Thomas's in London, Birmingham Women's and Children's Hospital and Solihull Hospital, and Glasgow Royal Hospital for Children and Glasgow Royal Infirmary in Scotland. We are full of gratitude for all you do for us, supporting us, getting us the treatments we need, and the thousands of letters you send to our GPs and other medical professionals to teach them about EB, and to explain that not everything to do with our health is linked to our EB.

Thanks must go to you, the reader, for being willing to learn more about this often brutal condition. Whether you are someone who lives with EB, are someone who knows someone with EB, are working with people with EB, or you're just curious, every person that reads this will be learning about the condition and raising awareness of it. Thank you.

And, finally, to the EB community, in the UK and globally, you are wonderful, you are strong, you are brave; thank you for being who you are.

www.debra.org.uk
www.cure-eb.org

Printed in Great Britain
by Amazon